I0483794

"It was easier to talk with my doctor after reading this booklet. And I was glad to learn that most breast changes are not cancer."

Table of Contents

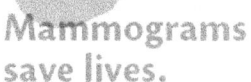

Mammograms save lives.

Mammograms are tests to check for breast changes that are often too small for you or your doctor to feel. If you are 40 or older, having a mammogram every 1 to 2 years could save your life. For information about free or low-cost mammograms, see pages 29 and 30.

To order free copies of this booklet, call the National Cancer Institute (NCI) at 1-800-4-CANCER (1-800-422-6237) or visit us online at www.cancer.gov.

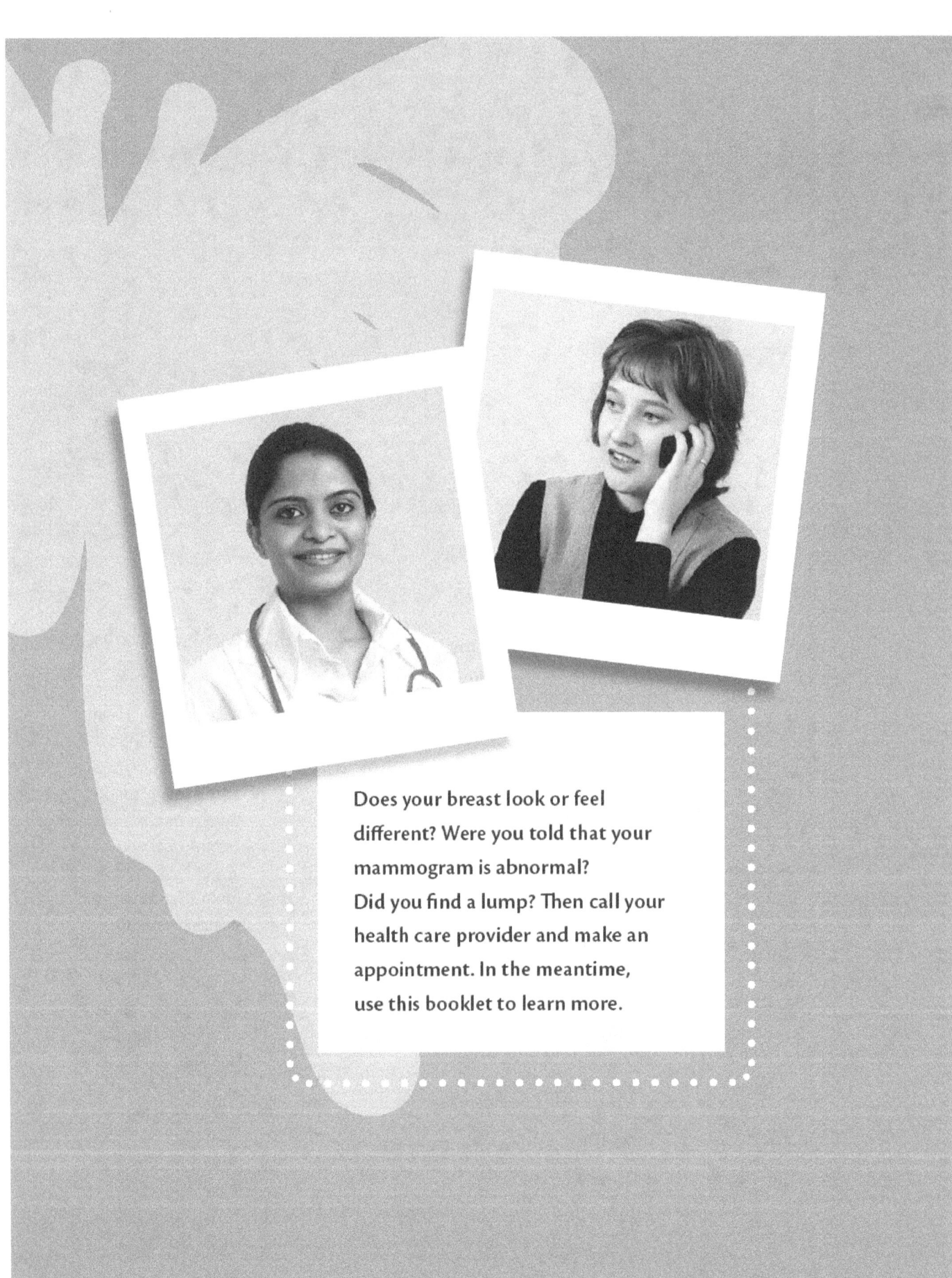

Does your breast look or feel different? Were you told that your mammogram is abnormal? Did you find a lump? Then call your health care provider and make an appointment. In the meantime, use this booklet to learn more.

Introduction

You may be reading this booklet because you, or your health care provider, found a **breast** lump or other breast change. Keep in mind that breast changes are very common. Most breast changes are not **cancer**. But it is very important to get the follow-up tests that your health care provider asks you to.

What are breast changes?

Many breast changes are changes in how your breast or **nipple** looks or feels. You may notice a lump or firmness in your breast or under your arm. Or perhaps the size or shape of your breast has changed. Your nipple may be pointing or facing inward (inverted) or feeling tender. The skin on your breast, **areola**, or nipple may be scaly, red, or swollen. You may have **nipple discharge**, which is an **abnormal** fluid coming from the nipple.

If you have these or other breast changes, talk with your health care provider to get these changes checked as soon as possible.

This booklet can help you take these steps:

- Call your health care provider to make an appointment as soon as you notice any breast changes.

- Go back to see your health care provider if your **mammogram** result is abnormal.

- Get all of the follow-up tests and care that your health care provider asks you to.

It may be helpful to bring this booklet with you. It discusses breast changes that are not cancer (**benign**), as well as changes that are abnormal or could be signs of cancer. Feel free to read different sections in this booklet as you need them. The *Words to know* section in the back of this booklet defines words that are shown in bold the first time they are used.

Anatomy of the breast

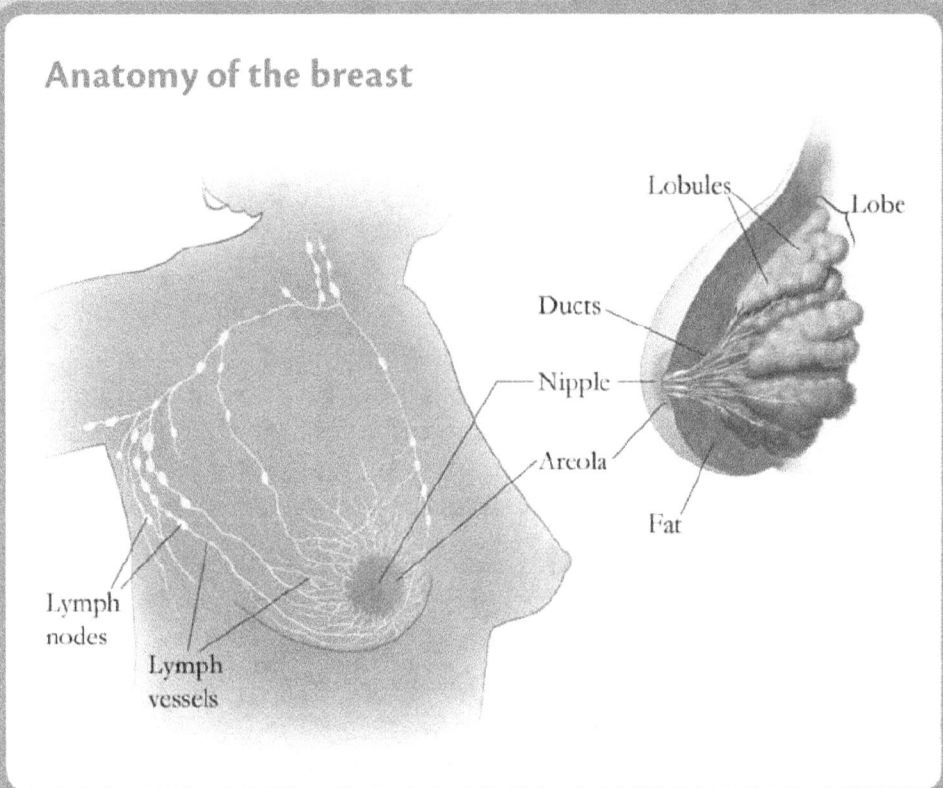

Lobules

Lobe

Ducts

Nipple

Areola

Fat

Lymph
nodes

Lymph
vessels

1 Breast and lymphatic system basics

To better understand breast changes, it helps to know what the breasts and **lymphatic system** are made of.

What are breasts made of?

Breasts are made of **connective tissue**, **glandular** tissue, and fatty tissue. Connective tissue and glandular tissue look dense, or white on a mammogram. Fatty tissue is non-dense, or black on a mammogram. **Dense breasts** can make mammograms harder to interpret.

Breasts have **lobes**, **lobules**, **ducts**, an areola, and a nipple.

- Lobes are sections of the glandular tissue. Lobes have smaller sections called lobules that end in tiny bulbs that can make milk.

- Ducts are thin tubes that connect the lobes and lobules. Milk flows from the lobules through the ducts to the nipple.

- The nipple is the small raised area at the tip of the breast. Milk flows through the nipple. The areola is the area of darker-colored skin around the nipple. Each breast also has **lymph vessels**.

What is the lymphatic system made of?

The lymphatic system, which is a part of your body's defense system, contains lymph vessels and lymph nodes.

- Lymph vessels are thin tubes that carry a fluid called **lymph** and **white blood cells**.

- Lymph vessels lead to small, bean-shaped organs called **lymph nodes**. Lymph nodes are found near your breast, under your arm, above your collarbone, in your chest, and in other parts of your body.

- Lymph nodes filter substances in lymph to help fight **infection** and disease. They also store disease-fighting white blood cells called **lymphocytes**.

2 Check with your health care provider about breast changes

Check with your health care provider if you notice that your breast looks or feels different. No change is too small to ask about. In fact, the best time to call is when you first notice a breast change.

Breast changes to see your health care provider about:

A lump (mass) or a firm feeling

◆ A lump in or near your breast or under your arm

◆ Thick or firm tissue in or near your breast or under your arm

◆ A change in the size or shape of your breast

Lumps come in different shapes and sizes. Most lumps are not cancer.

If you notice a lump in one breast, check your other breast. If both breasts feel the same, it may be normal. Normal breast tissue can sometimes feel lumpy.

Some women do monthly **breast self-exams (BSE)**. Doing a BSE can help you learn how your breast normally feels, and make it easier to notice and find any changes. Talk with your health care provider if you would like to learn more.

Remember—getting mammograms and having a **clinical breast exam** (an exam done by a health care provider) on a regular basis are the best ways to find breast cancer early in most women.

 Always get a lump checked. Don't wait until your next mammogram. You may need to have tests to be sure that the lump is not cancer.

Nipple discharge or changes

◆ Nipple discharge (fluid that is not breast milk)

◆ Nipple changes, such as a nipple that points or faces inward (inverted) into the breast

Nipple discharge may be different colors or textures. Nipple discharge is not usually a sign of cancer. It can be caused by birth control pills, some medicines, and infections.

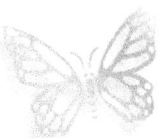 Get nipple discharge checked, especially fluid that comes out by itself or fluid that is bloody.

Skin changes

◆ Itching, redness, scaling, dimples, or puckers on your breast

 If the skin on your breast changes, get it checked as soon as possible.

"I was in the shower one morning, when I felt a small lump in my breast. I was afraid and busy, but I didn't let that stop me. I made an appointment to see my doctor. I got the answers I needed."

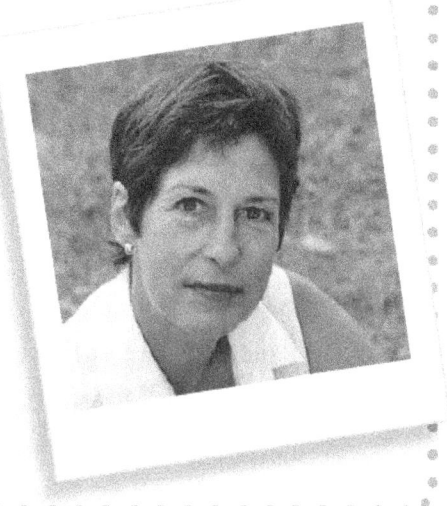

Talk with your health care provider.

To get the most from your visit, talk with your health care provider about any breast changes you notice, as well as your **personal medical history** and your **family medical history**.

Tell your health care provider about breast changes or problems:

◆ These are the breast changes or problems I have noticed: _____

◆ This is what the breast change looks or feels like: _____
(For example: Is the lump hard or soft? Does your breast feel tender or swollen? How big is the lump? What color is the nipple discharge?)

◆ This is where the breast change is: _____
(For example: What part of the breast feels different? Do both breasts feel different or only one breast?)

◆ This is when I first noticed the breast change: _____

◆ Since then, this is the change I've noticed: _____
(For example: Has it stayed the same or gotten worse?)

Share your personal medical history:

◆ I've had these breast problems in the past: _____

◆ These are the breast exams and tests that I have had: _____

◆ My last mammogram was on this date: _____

◆ My last menstrual period began on this date: _____

◆ These are the medicines or herbs that I take: _____

◆ Right now, I: ☐ Have breast implants ☐ Am pregnant ☐ Am breastfeeding

◆ I've had this type of cancer before: _____

Share your family medical history:

◆ My family members have had these breast problems or diseases: _____

◆ These family members had **breast cancer**: _____

◆ They were this old when they had breast cancer: _____

3 Breast changes during your lifetime that are not cancer

Most women have changes in their breasts during their lifetime. Many of these changes are caused by **hormones**. For example, your breasts may feel more lumpy or tender at different times in your **menstrual cycle**.

Other breast changes can be caused by the normal aging process. As you near **menopause**, your breasts may lose tissue and fat. They may become smaller and feel lumpy. Most of these changes are not cancer; they are called benign changes. However, if you notice a breast change, don't wait until your next mammogram. Make an appointment to get it checked.

Young women who have not gone through menopause often have more dense tissue in their breasts. Dense tissue has more glandular and connective tissue and less fat tissue. This kind of tissue makes mammograms harder to interpret—because both dense tissue and tumors show up as solid white areas on **x-ray** images. Breast tissue gets less dense as women get older.

Before or during your **menstrual periods**, your breasts may feel swollen, tender, or painful. You may also feel one or more lumps during this time because of extra fluid in your breasts. These changes usually go away by the end of your menstrual cycle. Because some lumps are caused by normal hormone changes, your health care provider may have you come back for a return visit, at a different time in your menstrual cycle.

During pregnancy, your breasts may feel lumpy. This is usually because the glands that produce milk are increasing in number and getting larger.

While breastfeeding, you may get a condition called **mastitis.** This happens when a milk duct becomes blocked. Mastitis causes the breast to look red and feel lumpy, warm, and tender. It may be caused by an infection and it is often treated with **antibiotics.** Sometimes the duct may need to be drained. If the redness or mastitis does not go away with treatment, call your health care provider.

As you approach menopause, your menstrual periods may come less often. Your hormone levels also change. This can make your breasts feel tender, even when you are not having your menstrual period. Your breasts may also feel more lumpy than they did before.

If you are taking hormones (such as **menopausal hormone therapy,** birth control pills, or injections) your breasts may become more dense. This can make a mammogram harder to interpret. Be sure to let your health care provider know if you are taking hormones.

When you stop having menstrual periods (menopause), your hormone levels drop, and your breast tissue becomes less dense and more fatty. You may stop having any lumps, pain, or nipple discharge that you used to have. And because your breast tissue is less dense, mammograms may be easier to interpret.

"I pay more attention to my breasts since my doctor did follow-up tests on changes that were found."

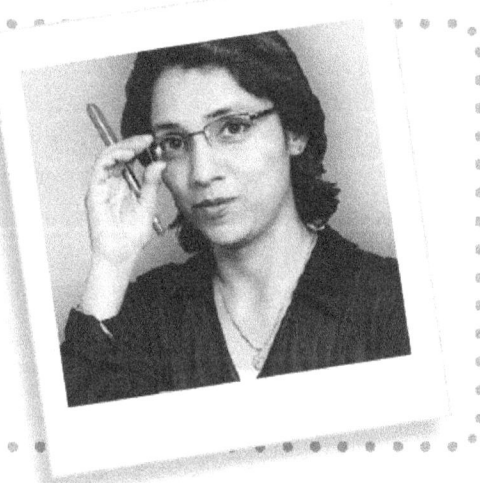

4 Finding breast changes

Here are some ways your health care provider can find breast changes:

Clinical breast exam

During a clinical breast exam, your health care provider checks your breasts and nipples and under your arms for any abnormal changes. This exam is part of a routine check-up. Some experts suggest that:

◆ Women in their 20s and 30s get a clinical breast exam every 3 years

◆ Women who are 40 and older get a clinical breast exam every year, as part of a routine check-up by a health care provider

Some women with a family history of breast cancer may need to have clinical breast exams and other screening tests more often.

Ask your health care provider at what age and how often you should have a clinical breast exam. During the visit, it's important to share your personal medical history and your family medical history. This includes problems or diseases that you or family members have had.

Mammogram

A mammogram is an x-ray picture of your breast tissue. This test may find tumors that are too small to feel. During a mammogram, each breast is pressed between two plastic plates. Some discomfort is normal, but if it's painful, tell the **mammography** technician.

The best time to get a mammogram is at the end of your menstrual period. This is when your breasts are less tender. Some women have less breast tenderness if they don't have any caffeine for a couple of days before the mammogram.

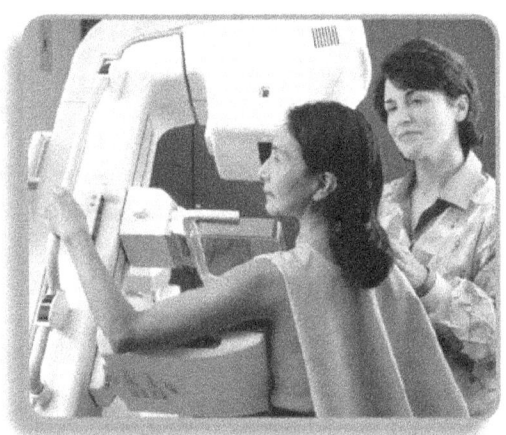

After the x-ray pictures are taken, they are sent to a **radiologist**, who studies them and sends a report to your health care provider.

Both film and digital mammography use x-rays to make a picture of the breast tissue. The actual procedure for getting the mammogram is the same. The difference is in how the images are recorded and stored. It's like the difference between a film camera and a digital camera.

◆ **Film mammography** stores the image directly on x-ray film.

◆ **Digital mammography** takes an electronic image of the breast and stores it directly in a computer. Digital images can be made lighter, darker, or larger. Images can also be stored and shared electronically.

A research study sponsored by the National Cancer Institute (NCI) showed that digital mammography and film mammography are about the same in terms of detecting breast cancer. However, digital mammography is better at detecting breast cancer in woman who are under age 50, have very dense breasts, or are **premenopausal** or **perimenopausal** (the times before and at the beginning of menopause).

Talk with your health care provider to learn more about what is best for you.

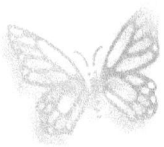

Women over age 40 should get a mammogram every 1 to 2 years. Women who are at increased risk of breast cancer should talk with their health care providers about whether to have mammograms before age 40 and how often to have them.

Mammograms are used for both screening and diagnosis.

◆ Screening mammogram

A **screening mammogram** is the kind of mammogram that most women get. It is used to find breast changes in women who have no signs of breast cancer.

◆ Diagnostic mammogram

If your recent screening mammogram found a breast change, or if a lump was found that needs to be checked, you may have a **diagnostic mammogram**. During a diagnostic mammogram, more x-ray pictures are taken to get views of the breast tissue from different angles. Certain areas of these pictures can also be made larger.

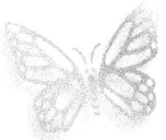

Talk with the women in your life. Let them know that mammograms save lives. Take time to care for yourself and those who need you.

"I'm glad to know that a test as simple and easy as a mammogram can find most breast changes early."

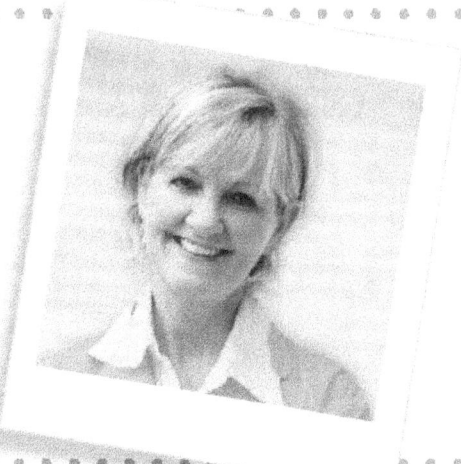

Mammograms and breast implants

When you make your appointment, be sure to tell the staff if you have **breast implants**. Ask if they have specialists who are trained in taking and reading mammograms of women with breast implants. This is important because breast implants can make it harder to see cancer or other abnormal changes on the mammogram. A special technique called **implant displacement views** is used.

- If you have breast implants for cosmetic reasons, you may have either a screening mammogram or a diagnostic mammogram. This will depend on the facility that does the mammogram.

- If you have breast implant(s) after having a **mastectomy** for breast cancer, talk with your breast **surgeon** or **oncologist** to learn about the best screening test for you.

MRI

Magnetic resonance imaging, also called **MRI**, uses a powerful magnet, radio waves, and a computer to take detailed pictures of areas inside the breast. MRI is another tool that can be used to find breast cancer. However, MRIs don't replace mammograms. They are used in addition to mammograms in women who are at increased risk of breast cancer.

MRIs have some limits. For example, they cannot find breast changes such as **microcalcifications**. MRIs are also less **specific** than other tests. This means that they may give **false-positive test results**—the test shows that there is cancer when there really is not.

Talk with your health care provider about having other screening tests, such as an MRI, in addition to mammograms. Ask your health care provider if you are at increased risk of breast cancer due to:

- Harmful changes (**mutations**) in the **BRCA1** or **BRCA2** gene
- A family history of breast cancer
- Your personal medical history

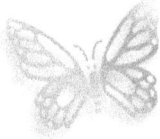

Keep in mind that MRIs are for women who are at increased risk of breast cancer.

5 Getting your mammogram results

You should get a written report of your mammogram results within 30 days of your mammogram, since this is the law. Be sure the mammography facility has your address and phone number. It's helpful to get your mammogram at the same place each year. This way, your current mammogram can be compared with past mammograms.

If your results were normal:

- Your breast tissue shows no signs of a **mass** or **calcification**.
- Visit your health care provider if you notice a breast change before your next appointment.

If your results were abnormal:

- A breast change was found. It may be benign (not cancer), **premalignant** (may become cancer), or cancer.
- It's important to get all the follow-up tests your health care provider asks you to.

If you don't get your results, call your health care provider.

Keep in mind that most breast changes are not cancer. But all changes need to be checked, and more tests may be needed.

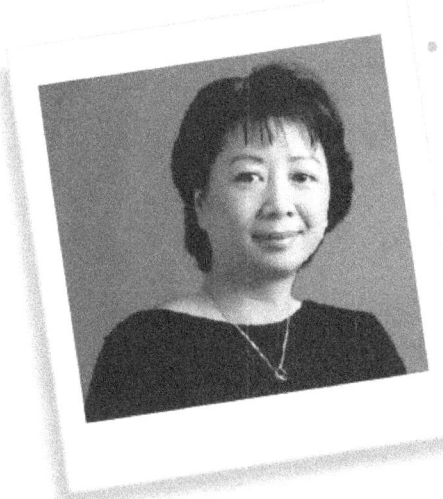

"I used to think when a mammogram found something, it was cancer. It turns out that most breast changes are *not* cancer. That's one thing I sure was glad to learn!"

What can a mammogram show?

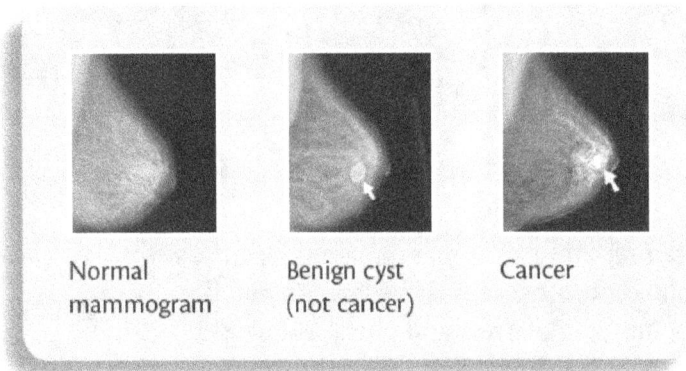

Normal mammogram   Benign cyst (not cancer)   Cancer

Mammograms can show lumps, **calcifications**, and other changes in your breast. The radiologist will study the mammogram for breast changes that do not look normal and for differences between your breasts. When possible, he or she will compare your most recent mammogram with past mammograms to check for changes.

Lump (or mass)

The size, shape, and edges of a lump give the radiologist important information. A lump that is not cancer often looks smooth and round and has a clear, defined edge. Lumps that look like this are often **cysts**. See page 20 for more information about cysts. However, if the lump on the mammogram has a jagged outline and an irregular shape, more tests are needed.

Depending on the size and shape of the lump, your health care provider may ask you to have:

- Another clinical breast exam

- Another mammogram to have a closer look at the area

- An **ultrasound** exam to find out if the lump is solid or is filled with fluid

- A test called a **biopsy** to remove cells, or the entire lump, to look at under a **microscope** to check for signs of disease

Calcifications

Calcifications are deposits of **calcium** in the breast tissue. They are too small to be felt, but can be seen on a mammogram. There are two types:

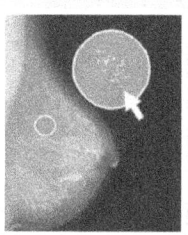

Calcium in your diet does not cause calcium deposits (calcifications) in the breast.

◆ **Macrocalcifications** look like small white dots on a mammogram. They are common in women over 50 years old. Macrocalcifications are not related to cancer and usually don't need more testing.

◆ **Microcalcifications** look like tiny white specks on a mammogram. They are usually not a sign of cancer. However, if they are found in an area of rapidly dividing cells, or grouped together in a certain way, you may need more tests.

Depending on how many calcifications you have, their size, and where they are found, your health care provider may ask you to have:

◆ Another mammogram to have a closer look at the area

◆ A test called a biopsy to check for signs of disease

Are mammogram results always right?

Mammography is an excellent tool to find breast changes in most women who have no signs of breast cancer. However, it may not detect all breast cancers. See your health care provider if you have a lump that was not seen on a mammogram or notice any other breast changes.

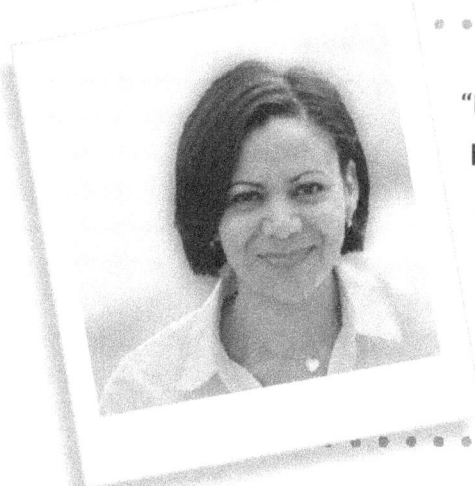

"Even though I was nervous, I'm glad I got the breast biopsy my doctor asked me to. As I waited for my results, it helped to remember the words of my doctor: 'Most breast changes are not cancer.' "

6 Follow-up tests to diagnose breast changes

An ultrasound exam, an MRI, a biopsy, or other follow-up tests may be needed to learn more about a breast change.

Ultrasound

An ultrasound exam uses sound waves to make a picture of breast tissue. This picture is called a **sonogram**. It helps radiologists to see if a lump or mass is solid or filled with fluid. A fluid-filled lump is called a cyst.

MRI

Magnetic resonance imaging, also called MRI, uses a powerful magnet, radio waves, and a computer to take detailed pictures of areas inside the breast. Sometimes breast lumps or large lymph nodes are found during a clinical breast exam or breast self-exam that were not seen on a mammogram or ultrasound. In these cases, an MRI can be used to learn more about these changes.

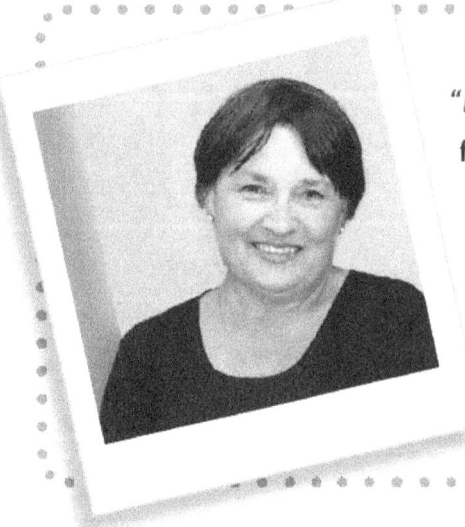

"My doctor said my mammogram found something 'abnormal.' That scared me, so I went back for more testing. It turned out that I had a benign cyst. It wasn't cancer. That was a relief."

Breast biopsy

A breast biopsy is a procedure to remove a sample of breast cells or tissue, or an entire lump. A **pathologist** then looks at the sample under a microscope to check for signs of disease. A biopsy is the only way to find out if cells are cancer.

Biopsies are usually done in an office or a clinic on an **outpatient** basis. This means you will go home the same day as the procedure. **Local anesthesia** is used for some biopsies. This means you will be awake, but you won't feel pain in your breast during the procedure. **General anesthesia** is often used for a **surgical biopsy**. This means that you will be asleep and won't wake up during the procedure.

Common types of breast biopsies:

◆ Fine-needle aspiration biopsy

A **fine-needle aspiration biopsy** is a simple procedure that takes only a few minutes. Your health care provider inserts a thin needle into the breast to take out fluid and cells.

◆ Core biopsy

A **core biopsy**, also called a core needle biopsy, uses a needle to remove small pieces or cores of breast tissue. The samples are about the size of a grain of rice. You may have a bruise, but usually not a scar.

◆ Vacuum-assisted biopsy

A **vacuum-assisted biopsy** uses a probe, connected to a vacuum device, to remove a small sample of breast tissue. The small cut made in the breast is much smaller than with surgical biopsy. This procedure causes very little scarring, and no stitches are needed.

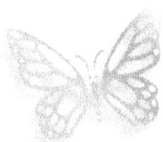

Your doctor may use ultrasound or mammography during a breast biopsy to help locate the breast change.

◆ Surgical biopsy

A surgical biopsy is an operation to remove part, or all, of a lump so it can be looked at under a microscope to check for signs of disease. Sometimes a doctor will do a surgical biopsy as the first step. Other times, a doctor may do a surgical biopsy if the results of a needle biopsy do not give enough information.

When only a sample of breast tissue is removed, it's called an **incisional biopsy**. When the entire lump or suspicious area is removed, it's called an **excisional biopsy**.

If the breast change cannot be felt, **wire localization**, also called **needle localization,** may be used to find the breast change. During wire localization, a thin, hollow needle is inserted into the breast. A mammogram is taken to make sure that the needle is in the right place. Then a fine wire is inserted through the hollow needle, to mark the area of tissue to be removed. Next, the needle is removed, and another mammogram is taken. You then go to the operating room where the surgeon removes the wire and surrounding breast tissue. The tissue is sent to the lab to be checked for signs of disease.

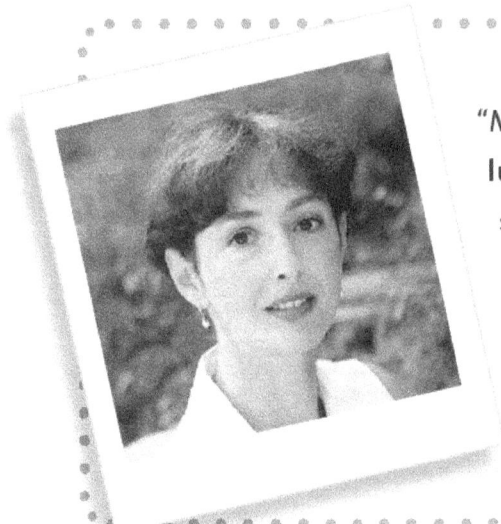

"My doctor found what felt like a lump during an exam. She said I should get a biopsy. I was afraid. But my doctor told me that it's always best to find out exactly what the problem is and take care of it early."

Questions to ask if a biopsy is recommended:

- Why is a biopsy needed? What will it tell us?_____
- What type of biopsy will I have? How will the biopsy be done? _____
- Where will the biopsy be done? How long will it take?_____
- Will it hurt? _____
- How much breast tissue will be removed?_____
- Will I be awake? _____
- What tests will be done on the breast tissue?_____
- When will I know the results?_____
- Will there be **side effects**?_____
- How should I care for the biopsy site? _____
- Will I need to rest after the biopsy? _____

Questions to ask about your biopsy results:

- What were the results of the biopsy? _____
- What do the biopsy results mean? _____
- What are the next steps? Do I need more tests? _____
- Who should I talk with next? _____
- Do I have an increased risk of breast cancer?_____
- Who can give me a second opinion on my biopsy results? _____

7 Breast changes and conditions: Getting follow-up test results

Test results will tell if you have:

Breast changes that are not cancer

These changes are not cancer and do not increase your risk of breast cancer. They are called benign changes.

Adenosis: Small, round lumps, or a lumpy feeling that are caused by enlarged breast lobules. Sometimes the lumps are too small to be felt. If there is scar-like tissue, the condition may be painful and is called **sclerosing adenosis**.

Cysts: Lumps filled with fluid. Breast cysts often get bigger and may be painful just before your menstrual period begins. Cysts are most common in premenopausal women and in women who are taking menopausal hormone therapy.

Fat necrosis: Round, firm lumps that usually don't hurt. The lumps most often appear after an injury to the breast, surgery, or radiation therapy.

Fibroadenomas: Hard, round lumps that may feel like a small marble and move around easily. They are usually painless and are most common in young women under 30 years old.

Intraductal papilloma: A wart-like growth in a milk duct of the breast. It's usually found close to the nipple and may cause clear, sticky, or bloody discharge from the nipple. It may also cause pain and a lump. It is most common in women 35–55 years old.

Ask your doctor when you will get your test results. See the chart on pages 25–28 for follow-up information.

Breast changes that are <u>not</u> cancer, but increase your risk of cancer

These conditions are not cancer, but having them increases your risk of breast cancer. They are considered **risk factors** for breast cancer. Other risk factors include, for example, your age and a family history of breast cancer.

- **Atypical hyperplasia:**

    - **Atypical lobular hyperplasia (ALH)** is a condition in which abnormal cells are found in the breast lobules.

    - **Atypical ductal hyperplasia (ADH)** is a condition in which abnormal cells are found in the breast ducts.

- **Lobular carcinoma in situ (LCIS)** is a condition in which abnormal cells are found in the breast lobules. There are more abnormal cells in the lobule with LCIS than with ALH. Since these cells have not spread outside the breast lobules, it's called "**in situ**," which is a Latin term that means "in place."

The abnormal cells found in these conditions are not cancer cells. If you have ALH, ADH, or LCIS, talk with a doctor who specializes in breast health to make a plan that works best for you. Depending on your personal and family medical history, it may include:

- Mammograms every year

- Clinical breast exams every 6 to 12 months

- **Tamoxifen** (for all women) or **raloxifene** (for postmenopausal women). These drugs have been shown to lower some women's risk of breast cancer.

- Surgery. A small number of women with LCIS and high risk factors for breast cancer may choose to have surgery.

- **Clinical trials**. Talk with your health care provider about whether a clinical trial is a good choice for you.

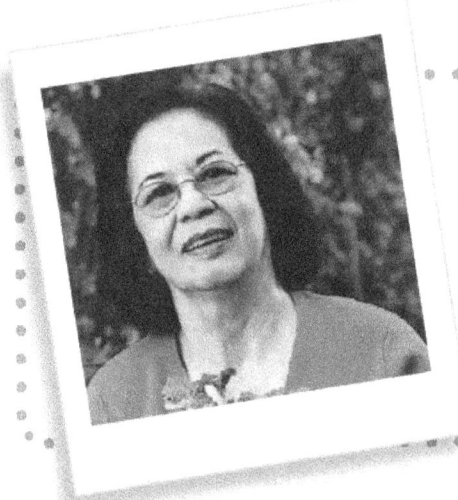

"Instead of stressing that something abnormal was found, I realized how lucky I was to have this small breast change found early."

Breast changes that may become cancer

Ductal carcinoma in situ (DCIS): DCIS is a condition in which abnormal cells are found in the lining of a breast duct. These cells have not spread outside the duct to the breast tissue. This is why it is called "in situ," which is a Latin term that means "in place." You may also hear DCIS called **Stage 0 breast carcinoma in situ** or **noninvasive** cancer.

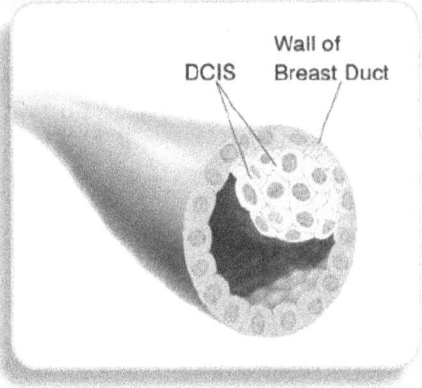

Since it's not possible to determine which cases of DCIS will become invasive breast cancer, it's important to get treatment for DCIS. Talk with a doctor who specializes in breast health to learn more. Treatment for DCIS is based on how much of the breast is affected, where DCIS is in the breast, and its **grade**. Most women with DCIS are cured with proper treatment.

Treatment choices for DCIS include:

- **Lumpectomy**. This is a type of **breast-conserving surgery** or **breast-sparing surgery**. It is usually followed by **radiation therapy**.

- Mastectomy. This type of surgery is used to remove the breast or as much of the breast tissue as possible.

- Tamoxifen. This drug may also be taken to lower the chance that DCIS will come back, or to prevent invasive breast cancer.

- Clinical trials. Talk with your health care provider about whether a clinical trial is a good choice for you.

Breast cancer

Breast cancer is a disease in which cancer cells form in the tissues of the breast. Breast cancer cells:

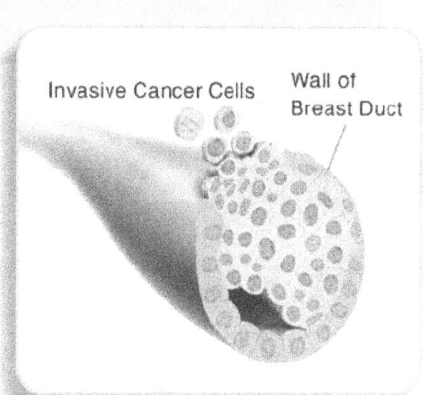

Invasive Cancer Cells | Wall of Breast Duct

- Grow and divide without control
- Invade nearby breast tissue
- May form a mass called a **tumor**
- May **metastasize**, or spread, to the lymph nodes or other parts of the body

After breast cancer has been **diagnosed**, tests are done to find out the extent, or **stage**, of the cancer. The stage is based on the size of the tumor and whether the cancer has spread. Treatment depends on the stage of the cancer.

For more information about breast cancer and to get answers to any questions you may have, call 1-800-4-CANCER (1-800-422-6237). Two free booklets you can ask for are: *What You Need To Know About Breast Cancer* and *Surgery Choices for Women with Early-Stage Breast Cancer*. You can also visit the National Cancer Institute (NCI) online at www.cancer.gov.

Get a second opinion

You may want to talk with another doctor to get a second opinion on your diagnosis or on your treatment. Many women do. And remember— it's important to talk with a doctor who specializes in breast cancer or in the breast condition that you have.

You can talk with your health care provider to find:

- Another pathologist to review your breast tissue slides and make a diagnosis
- Another surgeon, **radiation oncologist**, or **medical oncologist** to talk with about your treatment choices

Most doctors welcome a second opinion, especially when treatment is involved. Getting a second opinion is often covered, or even required, by your health insurance. Talking with another doctor can give you peace of mind. It can also help you make the best choices about your health.

8 Getting the support you need

It can be upsetting to notice a breast change, to get an abnormal test result, or to learn about a new condition or disease. We hope that the information in this booklet has answered some of your questions and calmed some of your fears as you talk with your health care provider and get the follow-up care you need.

Many women choose to get extra help and support for themselves. It may help to think about people who have been there for you during challenging times in the past.

◆ Ask friends or loved ones for support. Take someone with you while you are learning about your testing and treatment choices.

◆ Ask your health care provider to:

   ▪ Explain medical terms that are new or confusing

   ▪ Share with you how other people have handled the types of feelings that you are having

   ▪ Tell you about specialists that you can talk with to learn more

◆ Get in touch with the organizations listed on pages 29 and 30 to learn more.

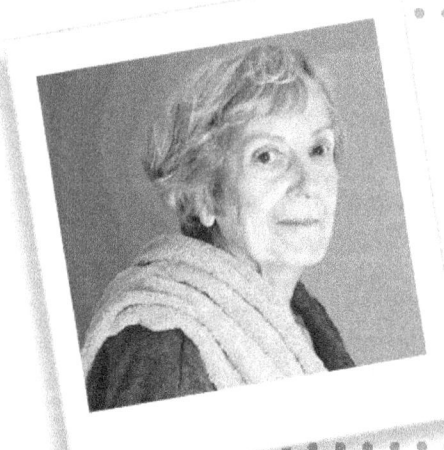

"I tried not to let the worries
of tomorrow bother me today.
It meant figuring out what
I could and could not control.
Talking with other women
helped me."

Breast conditions and follow-up care

Condition	Features	What your doctor may recommend
Adenosis	• Small round lumps, lumpiness, or you may not feel anything at all • Enlarged breast lobules • If there is scar-like fibrous tissue, the condition is called sclerosing adenosis. It may be painful. • Some studies have found that women with sclerosing adenosis may have a slightly increased risk of breast cancer.	• A core biopsy or a surgical biopsy may be needed to make a diagnosis.
Atypical lobular hyperplasia (ALH)	• Abnormal cells in the breast lobules • ALH increases your risk of breast cancer.	Regular follow-up, such as: • Mammograms • Clinical breast exams Treatment, such as: • Tamoxifen (for all women) or raloxifene (for postmenopausal women)
Atypical ductal hyperplasia (ADH)	• Abnormal cells in the breast ducts • ADH increases your risk of breast cancer.	Regular follow-up, such as: • Mammograms • Clinical breast exams Treatment, such as: • Tamoxifen (for all women) or raloxifene (for postmenopausal women)

continued on next page

Condition	Features	What your doctor may recommend
Breast cancer	• Cancer cells found in the breast, with a biopsy • A lump in or near your breast or under your arm • Thick or firm tissue in or near your breast or under your arm • A change in the size or shape of your breast • A nipple that's turned inward (inverted) into the breast • Skin on your breast that is itchy, red, scaly, dimpled, or puckered • Nipple discharge that is not breast milk	Treatment depends on the extent or stage of cancer. Tests are done to find out if the cancer has spread to others parts of your body. Treatment may include: • Surgery • **Chemotherapy** • Radiation therapy • **Hormonal therapy** • **Biological therapy** Clinical trials may be an option for you. Talk with your doctor to learn more.
Cysts	• Lumps filled with fluid • Often in both breasts • May be painful just before your menstrual period begins • Some cysts may be felt. Others are too small to be felt. • Most common in women 35–50 years old	• Cysts may be watched by your doctor over time, since they may go away on their own. • Ultrasound can show if the lump is solid or filled with fluid. • Fine needle aspiration may be used to remove fluid from the cyst.
Ductal carcinoma in situ (DCIS)	• Abnormal cells in the lining of a breast duct • Unlike cancer cells that can spread, these abnormal cells have not spread outside the breast duct. • May be called noninvasive cancer or Stage 0 breast carcinoma in situ.	Treatment is needed because doctors don't know which cases of DCIS may become invasive breast cancer. Treatment choices include: • Lumpectomy. This is a type of breast-conserving surgery or breast-sparing surgery. It is usually followed by radiation therapy. • Mastectomy. Surgery to remove the breast. • Tamoxifen. This drug may be taken to lower the chance that DCIS will come back after treatment or to prevent invasive breast cancer. • Clinical trials. Talk with your doctor about whether a clinical trial is a good choice for you. *continued on next page*

continued on next page

Condition	Features	What your doctor may recommend
Fat necrosis	• Round, firm lumps that usually don't hurt • May appear after an injury to the breast, surgery, or radiation therapy • Formed by damaged fatty tissue • Skin around the lump may look red, bruised, or dimpled • A benign (not cancer) breast condition	• A biopsy may be needed to diagnose and remove fat necrosis, since it often looks like cancer. • Fat necrosis does not usually need treatment.
Fibroadenoma	• Hard, round lumps that move around easily and usually don't hurt • Often found by the woman • Appear on a mammogram as smooth, round lumps with clearly defined edges • The most common benign breast tumors • Common in women under 30 years old • Most fibroadenomas do not increase your risk of breast cancer. However, complex fibroadenomas do slightly increase your risk.	• A biopsy may be needed to diagnose fibroadenoma. • A minimally invasive technique such as ultrasound-guided **cryoablation** or an excisional biopsy may be used to remove the lumps. • These growths may be watched by your doctor over time, since they may go away on their own.
Intraductal papilloma	• A wart-like growth inside the milk duct, usually close to the nipple • May cause pain and a lump • May cause clear, sticky, or bloody discharge • Most common in women 35–55 years old • Unlike single papillomas, multiple papillomas increase your risk of breast cancer.	• A biopsy may be needed to diagnose the growth and remove it.

continued on next page

Breast conditions and follow-up care continued

Condition	Features	What your doctor may recommend
Lobular carcinoma in situ (LCIS)	• A condition in which abnormal cells are found in the breast lobules • LCIS increases your risk of breast cancer.	Regular follow-up, such as: • Mammograms • Clinical breast exams Treatment choices: • Tamoxifen (for all women) or raloxifene (for postmenopausal women) may be taken. • A small number of women with LCIS and high risk factors for breast cancer may choose to have surgery. • Clinical trials may be an option for you. Talk with your doctor to learn more.
Macrocalcifications	• Calcium deposits in the breast that look like small white dots on a mammogram • Often caused by aging • Cannot be felt • Usually benign (not cancer) • Common in women over 50 years old	• Another mammogram may be needed to have a closer look at the area. • Treatment is usually not needed.
Microcalcifications	• Calcium deposits in the breast that look like tiny white specks on a mammogram • Not usually a sign of cancer. However, if found in an area of rapidly dividing cells or grouped together in a certain way, they may be a sign of DCIS or invasive breast cancer.	• Another mammogram or a biopsy may be needed to make a diagnosis.

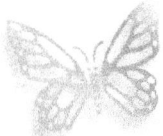

More information on these breast conditions can be found on www.cancer.gov or by calling 1-800-4-CANCER (1-800-422-6237).

Resources to learn more

National Cancer Institute (NCI)

NCI has comprehensive research-based information on cancer prevention, screening, diagnosis, treatment, genetics, and supportive care. We also have a clinical trials database and can offer tailored searches.

Phone: 1-800-4-CANCER (1-800-422-6237)

Web site: **www.cancer.gov** or **www.cancer.gov/espanol**

LiveHelp: **www.cancer.gov/livehelp**

Email: **cancergovstaff@mail.nih.gov**

Order publications at **www.cancer.gov/publications** or by calling 1-800-4-CANCER

We invite you to call or go online to talk with our trained information specialists, who speak English or Spanish, to:

◈ Get answers to any cancer-related questions you may have

◈ Get free NCI publications

◈ Learn more about specific resources and organizations in your area

◈ Find information on the NCI Web site **www.cancer.gov**

American Cancer Society (ACS)

ACS gives cancer information and support to patients, families, and caregivers. It also supports research, community education, advocacy, and public policy issues. Trained cancer information specialists can answer questions about cancer, link you to resources in your community, and provide information on local events.

Phone: 1-800-ACS-2345 (1-800-227-2345)

TTY: 1-866-228-4327

Web site: **www.cancer.org**

Centers for Disease Control and Prevention (CDC)

CDC conducts, supports, and promotes efforts to prevent cancer and increase early detection of cancer. CDC's National Breast and Cervical Cancer Early Detection Program (NBCCEDP) provides these services for underserved women:

◈ Clinical breast exams

◈ Mammograms (free or low-cost)

◈ Diagnostic tests if results are abnormal

◈ Referrals to treatment

Toll Free: 1-800-CDC-INFO (1-800-232-4636)

TTY: 1-888-232-6348

Web site: **www.cdc.gov**

Centers for Medicare & Medicaid Services (CMS)

CMS provides information for consumers about patient rights, prescription drugs, and health insurance issues, including Medicare and Medicaid.

Medicare is health insurance for people age 65 or older, under age 65 with certain disabilities, and any age with permanent kidney failure. It covers an annual screening mammogram, among other services. Medicare has information about providers in your area. English- or Spanish-speaking representatives can help you.

Phone: 1-800-MEDICARE (1-800-633-4227)

TTY: 1-877-486-2048

Web site: **www.cms.hhs.gov**

Medicaid is a program for people who need financial help with medical bills. You can learn more about this program by calling your local state welfare offices, state health department, state social services agencies, or your state's Medicaid office. Spanish-speaking staff is available in some offices.

Web site: **www.cms.hhs.gov**

National Women's Health Information Center (NWHIC)

NWHIC is a gateway to women's health information. NWHIC has English- and Spanish-speaking Information and Referral Specialists who will order free health information for you. They can also help you find organizations that can answer your health-related questions.

Phone: 1-800-994-9662

TDD: 1-888-220-5446

Web site: **www.womenshealth.gov**

U.S. Food and Drug Administration (FDA)

The FDA has fact sheets and brochures about mammography, as well as information about a certified mammography facility near you. It also has laws about how these facilities are run.

Phone: 1-888-INFO-FDA (1-888-463-6332)

Web site: **www.fda.gov**

Words to know

abnormal: Not normal. An abnormal lesion or growth may be cancer, premalignant (may become cancer), or benign (not cancer).

adenosis: A disease or abnormal change in a gland. Breast adenosis is a benign condition in which the lobules are larger than usual.

ADH (atypical ductal hyperplasia): A benign (not cancer) condition in which there are more cells than normal in the lining of breast ducts and the cells look abnormal under a microscope. Having ADH increases your risk of breast cancer.

ALH (atypical lobular hyperplasia): A benign (not cancer) condition in which there are more cells than normal in the breast lobules and the cells look abnormal under a microscope. Having ALH increases your risk of breast cancer.

antibiotic: A drug used to treat infections caused by bacteria and other microorganisms.

areola: The area of dark-colored skin on the breast that surrounds the nipple.

atypical hyperplasia: A benign (not cancer) condition in which cells look abnormal under a microscope and are increased in number.

benign: Not cancer. Benign tumors may grow larger but do not spread to other parts of the body.

biological therapy: Treatment to boost or restore the ability of the immune system to fight cancer, infections, and other diseases. Also used to lessen certain side effects that may be caused by some cancer treatments. Agents used in biological therapy include monoclonal antibodies, growth factors, and vaccines. These agents may also have a direct antitumor effect. Also called biological response modifier therapy, biotherapy, BRM therapy, and immunotherapy.

biopsy: The removal of cells or tissues for examination by a pathologist. The pathologist may study the tissue under a microscope or perform other tests on the cells or tissue. There are many different types of biopsy procedures. The most common types include: (1) incisional biopsy, in which only a sample of tissue is removed; (2) excisional biopsy, in which an entire lump or suspicious area is removed; and (3) needle biopsy, in which a sample of tissue or fluid is removed with a needle. When a wide needle is used, the procedure is called a core biopsy. When a thin needle is used, the procedure is called a fine-needle aspiration biopsy.

BRCA1: A gene on chromosome 17 that normally helps to suppress cell growth. A person who inherits certain mutations (changes) in a BRCA1 gene has a higher risk of getting breast, ovarian, prostate, and other types of cancer. BRCA1 is short for (**br**east **ca**ncer **1**, early onset gene).

BRCA2: A gene on chromosome 13 that normally helps to suppress cell growth. A person who inherits certain mutations (changes) in a BRCA2 gene has a higher risk of getting breast, ovarian, prostate, and other types of cancer. BRCA2 is short for (**br**east **ca**ncer **2**, early onset gene).

breast: Glandular organ located on the chest. The breast is made up of connective tissue, fat, and glandular tissue that can make milk. Also called mammary gland.

breast cancer: Cancer that forms in tissues of the breast, usually the ducts (tubes that carry milk to the nipple) and lobules (glands that make milk). It occurs in both men and women, although male breast cancer is rare.

breast density: Describes the relative amount of different tissues present in the breast. A dense breast has less fat than glandular and connective tissue. Mammogram films of breasts with higher density are harder to read and interpret than those of less dense breasts.

breast duct: A thin tube in the breast that carries milk from the breast lobules to the nipple. Also called milk duct.

breast implant: A silicone gel-filled or saline-filled sac placed under the chest muscle to restore breast shape.

breast-conserving surgery: An operation to remove the breast cancer but not the breast itself. Types of breast-conserving surgery include lumpectomy (removal of the lump), quadrantectomy (removal of one quarter, or quadrant, of the breast), and segmental mastectomy (removal of the cancer as well as some of the breast tissue around the tumor and the lining over the chest muscles below the tumor). Also called breast-sparing surgery.

breast self-exam: An exam by a woman of her breasts to check for lumps or other changes. Also called BSE.

breast-sparing surgery: An operation to remove the breast cancer but not the breast itself. Types of breast-sparing surgery include lumpectomy (removal of the lump), quadrantectomy (removal of one quarter, or quadrant, of the breast), and segmental mastectomy (removal of the cancer as well as some of the breast tissue around the tumor and the lining over the chest muscles below the tumor). Also called breast-conserving surgery.

calcification: Deposits of calcium in the tissues. Calcification in the breast can be seen on a mammogram, but cannot be felt. There are two types of breast calcifications, macrocalcification and microcalcification. Macrocalcifications are large deposits of calcium and are usually not related to cancer. Microcalcifications are specks of calcium that may be found in an area of rapidly dividing cells. Many microcalcifications clustered together may be a sign of cancer.

calcium: A mineral needed for healthy teeth, bones, and other body tissues. It is the most common mineral in the body. A deposit of calcium in body tissues, such as breast tissue, may be a sign of disease.

cancer: A term for diseases in which abnormal cells divide without control and can invade nearby tissues. Cancer cells can also spread to other parts of the body through the blood and lymph systems.

chemotherapy: Treatment with drugs that kill cancer cells.

clinical breast exam: A physical exam of the breast performed by a health care provider to check for lumps or other changes. Also called CBE.

clinical trial: A type of research study that tests how well new medical approaches work in people. A clinical trial tests new methods of screening, prevention, diagnosis, or treatment of a disease. Also called clinical study.

connective tissue: Supporting tissue that surrounds other tissues and organs. Specialized connective tissue includes bone, cartilage, blood, and fat.

core biopsy: The removal of a tissue sample with a wide needle for examination under a microscope. Also called core needle biopsy.

cryoablation: A procedure in which tissue is frozen to destroy abnormal cells. This is usually done with a special instrument that contains liquid nitrogen or liquid carbon dioxide. Also called cryosurgery.

cyst: A sac or capsule in the body. It may be filled with fluid or other material.

DCIS (ductal carcinoma in situ): A noninvasive condition in which abnormal cells are found in the lining of a breast duct. The abnormal cells have not spread outside the duct to other tissues in the breast. In some cases, DCIS may become invasive cancer and spread to other tissues, although it is not known at this time how to predict which lesions will become invasive. Also called intraductal carcinoma.

dense breasts: See breast density.

diagnosis: The process of identifying a disease, such as cancer, from its signs and symptoms.

diagnostic mammogram: X-ray of the breasts used to check for cancer after a lump or other sign or symptom of breast cancer has been found.

digital mammography: A technique that uses a computer, rather than x-ray film, to record x-ray images of the breast.

duct: See breast duct.

excisional biopsy: A surgical procedure in which an entire lump or suspicious area is removed for diagnosis. The tissue is then examined under a microscope to check for signs of disease.

false-positive test result: A test result that indicates that a person has a specific disease or condition when the person actually does not have the disease or condition.

family medical history: A record of the relationships among family members along with their medical histories. This includes current and past illnesses. A family medical history may show a pattern of certain diseases in a family. Also called family history.

fat necrosis: A benign condition in which fat tissue in the breast or other organs is damaged by injury, surgery, or radiation therapy. The fat tissue in the breast may be replaced by a cyst or by scar tissue, which may feel like a round, firm lump. The skin around the lump may look red, bruised, or dimpled.

fibroadenoma: A benign (not cancer) tumor that usually forms in the breast from both fibrous and glandular tissue. Fibroadenomas are the most common benign breast tumors.

film mammography: The use of x-rays to create a picture of the breast on a film.

fine-needle aspiration biopsy: The removal of tissue or fluid with a thin needle for examination under a microscope. Also called FNA biopsy.

general anesthesia: A temporary loss of feeling and a complete loss of awareness that feels like a very deep sleep. It is caused by special drugs or other substances called anesthetics. General anesthesia stops patients from feeling pain during surgery or other procedures.

gland: An organ that makes one or more substances, such as milk, hormones, digestive juices, sweat, tears, or saliva.

glandular: See gland.

grade: A description of a tumor based on how abnormal the cancer cells look under a microscope and how quickly the tumor is likely to grow and spread. Grading systems are different for each type of cancer.

hormonal therapy: Treatment that adds, blocks, or removes hormones. For certain conditions (such as diabetes or menopause), hormones are given to adjust low hormone levels. To slow or stop the growth of certain cancers (such as prostate and breast cancer), synthetic hormones or other drugs may be given to block the body's natural hormones. Sometimes surgery is needed to remove the gland that makes a certain hormone. Also called endocrine therapy, hormone therapy, and hormone treatment.

hormone: One of many chemicals made by glands in the body. Hormones circulate in the bloodstream and control the actions of certain cells or organs. Some hormones can also be made in the laboratory.

implant displacement views: A procedure used to do a mammogram (x-ray of the breasts) in women with breast implants. The implant is pushed back against the chest wall and the breast tissue is pulled forward and around it so the tissue can be seen in the mammogram. Also called Eklund displacement views and Eklund views.

in situ: In its original place. For example, in carcinoma in situ, abnormal cells are found only in the place where they first formed. They have not spread.

incisional biopsy: A surgical procedure in which a portion of a lump or suspicious area is removed for diagnosis. The tissue is then examined under a microscope to check for signs of disease.

infection: Invasion and multiplication of germs in the body. Infections can occur in any part of the body and can spread throughout the body. The germs may be bacteria, viruses, yeast, or fungi. They can cause a fever and other problems, depending on where the infection occurs. When the body's natural defense system is strong, it can often fight the germs and prevent infection. Some cancer treatments can weaken the natural defense system.

intraductal papilloma: A benign (not cancer), wart-like growth in a milk duct of the breast. It is usually found close to the nipple and may cause a discharge from the nipple. It may also cause pain and a lump in the breast that can be felt. It usually affects women aged 35-55 years. Having a single papilloma does not increase the risk of breast cancer. When there are multiple intraductal breast papillomas, they are usually found farther from the nipple. There may not be a nipple discharge and the papillomas may not be felt. Having multiple intraductal breast papillomas may increase the risk of breast cancer. Also called intraductal breast papilloma.

LCIS (lobular carcinoma in situ): A condition in which abnormal cells are found in the lobules of the breast. LCIS seldom becomes invasive cancer; however, having it in one breast increases the risk of developing breast cancer in either breast.

lobe: A portion of an organ, such as the breast, liver, lung, thyroid, or brain.

lobule: A small lobe or a subdivision of a lobe.

local anesthesia: A temporary loss of feeling in one small area of the body caused by special drugs or other substances called anesthetics. The patient stays awake but has no feeling in the area of the body treated with the anesthetic.

lumpectomy: Surgery to remove abnormal tissue or cancer from the breast and a small amount of normal tissue around it. It is a type of breast-sparing surgery.

lymph: The clear fluid that travels through the lymphatic system and carries cells that help fight infections and other diseases. Also called lymphatic fluid.

lymph node: A rounded mass of lymphatic tissue that is surrounded by a capsule of connective tissue. Lymph nodes filter lymph (lymphatic fluid), and they store lymphocytes (white blood cells). They are located along lymph vessels. Also called a lymph gland.

lymph vessel: A thin tube that carries lymph (lymphatic fluid) and white blood cells through the lymphatic system. Also called lymphatic vessel.

lymphatic system: The tissues and organs that produce, store, and carry white blood cells that fight infections and other diseases. This system includes the bone marrow, spleen, thymus, lymph nodes, and lymph vessels (a network of thin tubes that carry lymph and white blood cells). Lymph vessels branch, like blood vessels, into all the tissues of the body.

lymphocyte: A type of immune cell that is made in the bone marrow and is found in the blood and in lymph tissue. The two main types of lymphocytes are B lymphocytes and T lymphocytes. B lymphocytes make antibodies, and T lymphocytes help kill tumor cells and help control immune responses. A lymphocyte is a type of white blood cell.

macrocalcification: A small deposit of calcium in the breast that cannot be felt but can be seen on a mammogram. It is usually caused by aging, an old injury, or inflamed tissue and is usually not related to cancer.

mammogram: An x-ray of the breast.

mammography: The use of x-rays to create a picture of the breast tissue.

mass: In medicine, a lump in the body. It may be caused by the abnormal growth of cells, a cyst, hormonal changes, or an immune reaction. A mass may be benign (not cancer) or malignant (cancer).

mastectomy: Surgery to remove the breast, or as much of the breast tissue as possible.

mastitis: A condition in which breast tissue is inflamed. It is usually caused by an infection and is most often seen in nursing mothers.

medical oncologist: A doctor who specializes in diagnosing and treating cancer using chemotherapy, hormonal therapy, and biological therapy. A medical oncologist often is the main health care provider for someone who has cancer. A medical oncologist also gives supportive care and may coordinate treatment given by other specialists.

menopause: The time of life when a woman's ovaries stop working and menstrual periods stop. Natural menopause usually occurs around age 50. A woman is said to be in menopause when she hasn't had a period for 12 months in a row. Symptoms of menopause include hot flashes, mood swings, night sweats, vaginal dryness, trouble concentrating, and infertility.

menopausal hormone therapy: Hormones (estrogen, progesterone, or both) given to women after menopause to replace the hormones no longer produced by the ovaries. Also called hormone replacement therapy and HRT.

menstrual cycle: The monthly cycle of hormonal changes from the beginning of one menstrual period to the beginning of the next.

menstrual period: The periodic discharge of blood and tissue from the uterus. From puberty until menopause, menstruation occurs about every 28 days, but does not occur during pregnancy.

metastasize: To spread from one part of the body to another. When cancer cells metastasize and form secondary tumors, the cells in the metastatic tumor are like those in the original (primary) tumor.

microcalcification: A tiny deposit of calcium in the breast that cannot be felt but can be detected on a mammogram. A cluster of these very small specks of calcium may indicate that cancer is present.

microscope: An instrument that is used to look at cells and other small objects that cannot be seen with the eye alone.

MRI (magnetic resonance imaging): A procedure in which radio waves and a powerful magnet linked to a computer are used to create detailed pictures of areas inside the body. These pictures can show the difference between normal and diseased tissue. MRI makes better images of organs and soft tissue than other scanning techniques, such as computed tomography (CT) or x-ray. MRI is especially useful for imaging the brain, the spine, the soft tissue of joints, and the inside of bones. Also called NMRI and nuclear magnetic resonance imaging.

mutation: Any change in the DNA of a cell. Mutations may be caused by mistakes during cell division, or they may be caused by exposure to DNA-damaging agents in the environment. Mutations can be harmful, beneficial, or have no effect. If they occur in cells that make eggs or sperm, they can be inherited; if mutations occur in other types of cells, they are not inherited. Certain mutations may lead to cancer or other diseases.

needle localization: A procedure used to mark a small area of abnormal tissue so it can be removed by surgery. An imaging device is used to guide a thin wire with a hook at the end through a hollow needle to place the wire in or around the abnormal area. Once the wire is in the right place, the needle is removed and the wire is left in place so the doctor will know where the abnormal tissue is. The wire is removed at the time the biopsy is done. Also called needle/wire localization and wire localization.

nipple: In anatomy, the small raised area in the center of the breast through which milk can flow to the outside.

nipple discharge: Fluid coming from the nipple that is not breast milk.

noninvasive: In cancer, it describes disease that has not spread outside the tissue in which it began. In medicine, it describes a procedure that does not require inserting an instrument through the skin or into a body opening.

oncologist: A doctor who specializes in treating cancer. Some oncologists specialize in a particular type of cancer treatment. For example, a radiation oncologist specializes in treating cancer with radiation.

outpatient: A patient who visits a health care facility for diagnosis or treatment without spending the night. Sometimes called a day patient.

pathologist: A doctor who identifies diseases by studying cells and tissues under a microscope.

perimenopausal: Describes the time in a woman's life when menstrual periods become irregular as she approaches menopause. This is usually three to five years before menopause and is often marked by many of the symptoms of menopause, including hot flashes, mood swings, night sweats, vaginal dryness, trouble concentrating, and infertility.

personal medical history: A collection of information about a person's health. It may include information about allergies, illnesses and surgeries, and dates and results of physical exams, tests, screenings, and immunizations. It may also include information about medicines taken and about diet and exercise. Also called personal health record and personal history.

premalignant: A term used to describe a condition that may (or is likely to) become cancer. Also called precancerous.

premenopausal: Having to do with the time before menopause. Menopause ("change of life") is the time of life when a woman's menstrual periods stop permanently.

radiation oncologist: A doctor who specializes in using radiation to treat cancer.

radiation therapy: The use of high-energy radiation from x-rays, gamma rays, neutrons, protons, and other sources to destroy cancer cells and shrink tumors. Radiation may come from a machine outside the body (external-beam radiation therapy), or it may come from radioactive material placed in the body near cancer cells (internal radiation therapy).

radiologist: A doctor who specializes in creating and interpreting pictures of areas inside the body. The pictures are produced with x-rays, sound waves, or other types of energy.

raloxifene: The active ingredient in a drug used to reduce the risk of invasive breast cancer in postmenopausal women who are at high risk of the disease or who have osteoporosis. It is also used to prevent and treat osteoporosis in postmenopausal women. It is also being studied in the prevention of breast cancer in certain premenopausal women and in the prevention and treatment of other conditions. Raloxifene blocks the effects of the hormone estrogen in the breast and increases the amount of calcium in bone. It is a type of selective estrogen receptor modulator (SERM).

risk factor: Something that may increase the chance of developing a disease. Some examples of risk factors for cancer include age, a family history of certain cancers, use of tobacco products, certain eating habits, obesity, lack of exercise, exposure to radiation or other cancer-causing agents, and certain genetic changes.

sclerosing adenosis: A benign condition in which scar-like tissue is found in a gland, such as the breast lobules or the prostate. A biopsy may be needed to tell the difference between the abnormal tissue and cancer. Women with sclerosing adenosis of the breast may have a slightly increased risk of breast cancer.

screening: Checking for disease when there are no symptoms. Since screening may find diseases at an early stage, there may be a better chance of curing the disease. Examples of cancer screening tests are the mammogram (breast), colonoscopy (colon), Pap smear (cervix), and PSA blood level and digital rectal exam (prostate). Screening can also include checking for a person's risk of developing an inherited disease by doing a genetic test.

screening mammogram: X-rays of the breasts taken to check for breast cancer in the absence of signs or symptoms.

side effect: A problem that occurs when treatment affects healthy tissues or organs. Some common side effects of cancer treatment are fatigue, pain, nausea, vomiting, decreased blood cell counts, hair loss, and mouth sores.

sonogram: A computer picture of areas inside the body created by bouncing high-energy sound waves (ultrasound) off internal tissues or organs. Also called an ultrasonogram.

specific: See specificity.

specificity: When referring to a medical test, specificity refers to the percentage of people who test negative for a specific disease among a group of people who do not have the disease. No test is 100% specific because some people who do not have the disease will test positive for it (false positive).

stage: The extent of a cancer in the body. Staging is usually based on the size of the tumor, whether lymph nodes contain cancer, and whether the cancer has spread from the original site to other parts of the body.

stage 0 breast carcinoma in situ: There are 2 types of stage 0 breast cancer: ductal carcinoma in situ (DCIS) and lobular carcinoma in situ (LCIS). DCIS is a noninvasive condition in which abnormal cells are found in the lining of a breast duct (a tube that carries milk to the nipple). The abnormal cells have not spread outside the duct to other tissues in the breast. In some cases, DCIS may spread to other tissues, although it is not known how to predict which lesions will become invasive cancer. LCIS is a condition in which abnormal cells are found in the lobules (small sections of tissue involved with making milk) of the breast. This condition seldom becomes invasive cancer; however, having LCIS in one breast increases the risk of developing breast cancer in either breast. Stage 0 breast cancer is also called breast carcinoma in situ.

surgeon: A doctor who removes or repairs a part of the body by operating on the patient.

surgery: A procedure to remove or repair a part of the body or to find out whether disease is present. Also called an operation.

surgical biopsy: The removal of tissue by a surgeon for examination by a pathologist. The pathologist may study the tissue under a microscope.

tamoxifen: A drug used to treat certain types of breast cancer in women and men. It is also used to prevent breast cancer in women who have had (DCIS) ductal carcinoma in situ (abnormal cells in the ducts of the breast) and women who are at a high risk of developing breast cancer. Tamoxifen is also being studied in the treatment of other types of cancer. It blocks the effects of the hormone estrogen in the breast. Tamoxifen is a type of antiestrogen. Also called tamoxifen citrate.

tumor: An abnormal mass of tissue that results when cells divide more than they should or do not die when they should. Tumors may be benign (not cancer), or malignant (cancer). Also called neoplasm.

ultrasound: A procedure in which high-energy sound waves are bounced off internal tissues or organs and make echoes. The echo patterns are shown on the screen of an ultrasound machine, forming a picture of body tissues called a sonogram. Also called ultrasonography.

vacuum-assisted biopsy: A procedure in which a small sample of tissue is removed from the breast. An imaging device is used to guide a hollow probe connected to a vacuum device. The probe is inserted through a tiny cut made in numbed skin on the breast. The tissue sample is removed using gentle vacuum suction and a small rotating knife within the probe. Then the tissue sample is studied under a microscope to check for signs of disease. This procedure causes very little scarring and no stitches are needed. Also called VACB and vacuum-assisted core biopsy.

white blood cell: A type of immune cell. Most white blood cells are made in the bone marrow and are found in the blood and lymph tissue. White blood cells help the body fight infections and other diseases. Granulocytes, monocytes, and lymphocytes are white blood cells. Also called leukocyte and WBC.

wire localization: A procedure used to mark a small area of abnormal tissue so it can be removed by surgery. An imaging device is used to guide a thin wire with a hook at the end through a hollow needle to place the wire in or around the abnormal area. Once the wire is in the right place, the needle is removed and the wire is left in place so the doctor will know where the abnormal tissue is. The wire is removed when a biopsy is done. Also called needle localization and needle/wire localization.

x-ray: A type of high-energy radiation. In low doses, x-rays are used to diagnose diseases by making pictures of the inside of the body. In high doses, x-rays are used to treat cancer.

www.ingramcontent.com/pod-product-compliance
Lightning Source LLC
Chambersburg PA
CBHW081404170526

45166CB00010B/3200